All Natural Dental Remedies

Herbs and Home Remedies to Heal Your Teeth & Naturally Restore Tooth Enamel

Angela Kaelin

2012
Winter Tempest Books

ISBN-10: 0615719368
ISBN-13: 978-0615719368
Winter Tempest Books

DEDICATION

In memory of my grandparents.

CONTENTS

INTRODUCTION

This book supplies information about home remedies for the teeth and gums. It is not a medical book nor is it intended to be a substitute for allopathic medical or dental care when it is really needed.

It does not purport to show how to regenerate lost teeth. Although, the possibility of regrowing teeth seems greater once you understand that teeth are tissue like any other tissue in the body. In fact, some successful experiments in this regard have been reported on animals by the University of Alberta, Canada involving the use of low intensity pulsed ultrasound (LIPUS) to stimulate the growth of the teeth. See: www.lipus.org. This procedure is still theoretical and not something the average person can make practical use of at this time.

This book is intended only to provide practical information about nutrition and specific herbal and mineral therapies, most of them from folk medicine, about how to heal the teeth and gums, which you can easily get your hands on and everyone can use.

There is nothing mysterious or mystical about

re-mineralizing teeth and naturally restoring tooth enamel. Yet, despite the renaissance of information about other aspects of natural healing, natural dental care is a subject that has not been much discussed. This is partly because to talk about natural dental enamel growth or healing of cavities is heresy against the official dental establishment. And, it is partly because when people believe there is no solution to a problem, they don't bother to look for one.

The purpose of "All Natural Dental Remedies" is not to make an argument for alternative dentistry or against conventional dentistry; nor is it to persuade anyone that one way of doing things is superior to another. Rather, it is to present practical information about the health and healing of the teeth and gums in a matter-of-fact way for informational purposes.

The types of remedies presented include nutritional, herbal, mineral and other alternative remedies. Unfortunately, there is very little mainstream scientific research on alternative dental remedies, so we must rely largely on folklore and what is called "anecdotal" evidence.

1 BASIC DEFINITIONS OF SOME TERMS AND SOME GENERAL CAUTIONS

The following are basic definitions used throughout this book:

Poultice: An application of a moist substance such as crushed herbs.

Infusion or Tea: A drink made by bringing water to a boil, then removing it from the heat and adding herbs in order to extract their active constituents by allowing them to steep for three to five minutes before straining.

Tincture: An extract of an herb in a solution of grain alcohol. Some commercially available tinctures use a non-alcoholic base.

Essential Oil: The volatile oils of a plant.

Decoction: A concentrated form of an infusion in which the herb is boiled until some of the water evaporates.

Tooth Powders: A dentifrice made by crushing and pulverizing herbs and other ingredients. To use a tooth powder, moisten a soft toothbrush, dip it into the powder and gently brush your teeth.

General Warning Regarding the Use of Herbs and Essential Oils

Care has been taken to, as much as possible, exclude herbs, which might pose the most risk to sensitive people, however, any herb may pose risks to people who have allergies, whose health is delicate or who are taking pharmaceutical drugs.

Horsetail (Equisetum arvense), when it is used strictly as a dentifrice where it is spat out or in homeopathic form, should pose no or low risk. But, it should not be ingested by pregnant or nursing women, men suffering from prostate cancer or anyone who has a pre-existing liver or bladder condition or who is taking pharmaceutical drugs called ACE inhibitors.

If you are under the care of a physician, especially for liver disease, kidney disease, high blood pressure or cardiac disease, you should consult with your doctor before taking this or any other herb. Horsetail should be used only in recommended amounts and usage of the herb should not exceed ten days at a time after which you should take, at least, a three day break. If you experience any urinary tract infections or kidney or bladder related discomfort, discontinue the use of the herb immediately.

Chaparral root should not be ingested by people who have pre-existing liver conditions. This herb is no longer available in Canada.

Horsetail and chaparral are both considered "poisonous plants" by the Food and Drug Administration in the U.S.

These herbs used solely as a dentifrice and not swallowed should not present a danger. Homeopathic versions of the herbs pose no risk.

Valerian root is generally considered safe, however, you should take caution with valerian, if you are prone to seizures, epilepsy, liver failure, cirrhosis of the liver, hepatitis, are pregnant or breastfeeding and, as always, if you are under the care of a physician, you should ask him or her before taking any supplements or herbs, especially, if you are taking pharmaceutical drugs.

Many essential oils should not be swallowed. Essential oils should never be used on babies or cats. Let common sense prevail in the use of all herbs and essential oils.

The quality of the herbs and essential oils you use is very important to their efficacy. Choose high-quality organic herbs.

When choosing essential oils, choose in favor of organic, food grade oils. Never use fragrance oils because these are artificial chemicals, whereas, essential oils are the extracted oils of the plant. Some essential oils are highly diluted with jojoba oil (another essential oil) and labeled "100% essential oil." The statement is true, but the extract of the particular herb may be very diluted and weakened. Let your senses be your guide when choosing essential oils and look for the purest extracts.

Where supplements are suggested, as a general rule, follow the recommended dosages and any warnings on the bottle.

What to Avoid

If you are trying to heal your teeth and gums or simply maintain good oral health, try to avoid the following:

Cigarette smoking may contribute to gum diseases by compromising the health of gum tissue, so for healthy gums, don't smoke.

Avoid mouthwashes or toothpastes containing sodium fluoride (toxic), sodium laurel sulfate (damages tissues) and glycerin (coats teeth and prevents healing).

2 PROPER NUTRITION IS THE FOUNDATION OF DENTAL HEALTH

Nutrition is at the foundation of healthy teeth. This was demonstrated most perfectly by Dr. Weston A. Price, who researched the dental health of people throughout the word and concluded that civilization was not good for people's teeth.

In 1939, he published the book, "Nutrition and Physical Degeneration: A Comparison of Primitive and Modern Diets and Their Effects," in which he demonstrated that the best diet for good dental health was a very traditional, if not primitive, one.

According to Dr. Price, refined sugar and processed grains should be rejected in favor of more natural, raw, unprocessed whole foods. Furthermore, more traditional diets that include soups made with broth of animal and fish stock help people to have healthier teeth and bones. The fish head soup of Thailand and traditional menudo soup of Mexico are examples of food that helps the health of the teeth because it contains nutrients similar to those from which the tissues of the teeth are constructed.

Eat soup made from scratch. Make your own broth and include tissue from the bones, the marrow, joints and cartilage.

Instead of processed foods and fast food, choose:

Whole grains such as spelt and oats
Canned fish like salmon and mackerel, which contain edible bones
Fish oil
Organic, raw dairy products
The juice of leafy green vegetables

Caution: Some people have reported a darkening of their teeth after eating a lot of fresh green vegetables. Instead, get the most nutrients out of your vegetables by juicing them.

Good juicing vegetables for dental health include:

Carrots
Spinach
Turnips, including the tops
Dandelion, including the leaves and the root
Lettuce

Get a quality juicer and start out slowly drinking the juice. If your body is highly toxic, you may find that you are only able to consume a few ounces at a time without feeling dizzy, headachey or sick. This is called the Herxheimer Effect and it can happen when you begin a detoxification program. Just go slowly, at first. Persevere and little by little, you will find that your body craves the juice. Always make it fresh and drink it as soon as you can. Feel free to experiment with your own recipes. There is no right or wrong way to make or consume raw juices.

Protect your teeth (and bones) from harmful chemicals in the water and food by taking an iodine supplement from dulse kelp like New Horizon's Sea-Adine.

Include kelp and bone meal in your diet along with the following vitamins and other nutrients to maintain and restore the health of the teeth and facilitate re-mineralization.

Vitamins and Other Nutrients

Bioflavinoids (Vitamin P)
B-Complex
B12
C (natural sources - do not chew)
CoQ10
D
E (natural sources)
K, especially K2
Magnesium

Silica, phosphorus and calcium all help with the repair of bone tissues. The trace minerals boron and selenium are, also, part of a diet for healthy teeth.

3 NATURAL REMEDIES FOR DENTAL PAIN

It goes without saying that dental pain is the symptom of another problem, however, if you are in pain, your first concern will be to put an end to it as quickly as possible. There are many remedies for the relief of painful teeth, some of which you may have in your kitchen cupboard, already.

Here is a list of common remedies from folklore:

Dissolve sea salt thoroughly in warm water and gently rinse your mouth with it.

Place a whole clove on the tooth or drop clove oil on a cotton ball and hold it against the affected area.

Other essential oils that can be used in a similar way are cajeput, caraway, chamomile, marjoram, wild Mediterranean oregano, peppermint and thyme oils. Always look for food grade oils.

Place a poultice of comfrey or lavender (or a warm comfrey or lavender tea bag) over the toothache.

Apply tarragon oil to the affected tooth or gently chew a few tarragon leaves and apply them as a poultice.

Place a few drops of vanilla extract (not imitation flavoring) on a cotton ball and apply it to the affected tooth.

Apply several drops of echinacea tincture to the tooth.

This is one of the best remedies for aching teeth: Take about 1/4 teaspoon of bentonite clay and 1/4 teaspoon of activated charcoal powder. Place it in a bowl or in the palm of your hand. Add several drops of colloidal silver to make a paste and apply it to the painful tooth. Caution: Do not use this on a broken tooth. This is especially powerful when it is done right before going to sleep.

Excruciating tooth pain can be caused by sinus congestion. Try to find relief by alternating hot and cold compresses until the pain stops. Applying a topical ointment like Tiger Balm to the skin can bring relief, as can inhaling very pure peppermint oil.

Also, see "Chapter 5 Oil Pulling" and "Chapter 7 Remedies for TMJ and Bruxism." "Bruxism" or tooth grinding" is another cause of dental pain.

4. HEALING THE GUMS

If you have problem gums, the medical term for which is "periodontal disease," you should begin the healing process of your teeth by healing your gums first. Diseased gums can lead to loose and lost teeth and it is related to other health problems, most notably a higher risk for cardiovascular disease.

General Remedies for Diseased Gums

After dental infections, gum disease is the main cause of loss of dental bone, so you should take care to eat a traditional diet including real soup broth with the bones and ligaments in it, soft fish bones and bone meal.

In a 1974 study, researchers noted that subjects who suffered from periodontal disease were also deficient in the enzyme CoQ10 (Nakamura 71). This was not the first study of its kind. A similar study was conducted on U.S. soldiers during World War II with a similar conclusion. Depletion of CoQ10, which is present in every cell of the body in a healthy person, is associated with aging.

There is no established dosage for CoQ10, although 30 to 90 mg per day is considered therapeutic. Other trials indicate it may be more effective at up to 1200 mg per day in divided does.

The herbs bilberry and hawthorn berry are known to generally strengthen the gum tissue.

A tea made of a small handful of parsley, held in the mouth and drunk slowly, is an old remedy for gum disease.

Another powerful remedy for all kinds of oral disease and pain is to take a swig of 10 to 15 ppm pure colloidal silver and hold it in your mouth for, at least, 5 to 6 minutes. Colloidal silver is a powerful natural antibiotic and cell rejuvenator. You can make a flavored mouthwash with colloidal silver by adding a few drops of peppermint oil.

In cases involving oral infections, colloidal silver is an excellent antibiotic. There is no established dosage for colloidal silver, however, in the case of infection, an adult might take 2 to 4 ounces per day in divided doses.

Colloidal silver is also an excellent remedy for monilia, thrush or oral candida.

Rinsing the mouth and brushing with food grade hydrogen peroxide is an excellent natural treatment for a variety of oral diseases. In acute cases, rinse your mouth two or three times per day.

Different Types of Gum Disease and Their Remedies

Swelling of the gums is usually indicative of another condition, such as abscesses, gingivitis or pyorrhea. It should not be taken lightly because, more rarely, it can be a symptom of more serious disease.

Abscesses

Abscesses can occur as a result of injury or infection in the gums. An abscess is a pus filled pocket, usually on the gums outside a tooth, which is also affected by the infection or which may actually be the source of infection. Untreated, an abscess could lead to the loss of a tooth as well as a fever because the infection can spread throughout the entire body.

Apply any of the following oils to a piece of cotton ball and lay it next to the abscess: Neem oil; clove oil; tea tree oil; or wild Mediterranean oregano oil. Neem oil is especially healing to the gums. It has a very bitter taste, but, if you are in pain, you probably won't care.

To fight infection and fever, use colloidal silver or wild Mediterranean oregano orally.

Combine these treatments with oil pulling. See "Chapter 5 Oil Pulling."

Gingivitis (Infection of the Gums)

The primary herb, traditionally used in the treatment of gingivitis, is myrrh. A tincture of myrrh, essential oil of myrrh or myrrh tea should be applied to the teeth and gums three times per day until the problem subsides. Hold the myrrh in your mouth as long as possible after an application. After that, apply once per day to maintain gum health.

Supplement your diet with Vitamin C and bioflavinoids. This is the nutritional support infected gums need.

A Simple, Highly Effective Myrrh Mouthwash

1/2 cup vodka or brandy
20 myrrh capsules
1/2 cup warm water

Empty the myrrh capsules into the warm water and stir until dissolved. When it is cool, add vodka or brandy. Mix thoroughly and bottle as a mouthwash. Use this three times per day for an acute case of gingivitis.

A Simple Clove Oil Remedy

Add approximately 10 drops of clove oil to an ounce of olive oil, sesame seed or other edible oil. Mix these two ingredients together and apply the oil to your gums with a Q-tip or a cotton ball three times per day until you find relief.

Herbal Remedy for Gingivitis

This is a natural remedy to stop gingivitis, toothaches and mouth sores. It works to prevent gingivitis, as well.

1/2 cup turmeric, ground
1/2 cup myrrh, powdered
1/2 cup dried peppermint leaves, ground
1/4 cup cinnamon, ground
A pinch of cloves, ground

Mix all ingredients thoroughly and apply as a tooth powder, dipping your toothbrush into it and gently brushing your teeth. If you have gingivitis, brush with this formula three times per day. After brushing, spit out the saliva, but do not rinse your mouth.

Pockets in the Gums

Apply bayberry tincture to the gums. This is a fast-acting astringent that will help tighten up the gum tissue.

Neem oil is another fast-acting natural antibiotic, which will soothe gums and help them heal very quickly.

Put a cup of colloidal silver into an oral irrigator (Waterpik device) and use it on a low setting. Do not rinse your mouth.

You may also add oils such as spearmint, peppermint, clove and other gum healers to the reservoir, but when you're finished, clean the oils out of the machine by running pure warm water and a few drops of vinegar through the machine.

Do this twice per day until your gums heal and tighten.

Use any of the following astringent herbs in the form of poultices or tinctures, in tooth powders or as rinses for the mouth:

Bayberry
Neem or margosa (very powerful for healing gums quickly)
Banyan tree bark
Prickly ash bark
Turmeric root
Echinacea root

Receding Gums

Always brush your teeth gently with a soft toothbrush to avoid causing injury and damage to your gums. As long as your gums are not sore, swollen, abscessed or otherwise painful or diseased, you should massage them for a minute or two with your clean fingers after brushing. Do this with the idea that you are "re-forming" the gums and pulling them down over the teeth where they belong.

Chamomile, cinnamon, echinacea and hawthorn berries made into teas or tinctures help the healing of the gums and work to reduce inflammation.

Receding gums can be symptomatic of gingivitis.

Pyorrhea
(Pus-filled Decaying Gums)

Grind dried holy basil leaves and use them as a tooth powder. If you like, include powdered sage leaves, myrrh and goldenseal.

Make a tincture or tea of any of these herbs and rinse your mouth three times per day.

Pyorrhea Remedy

2 ounces echinacea tincture
30 drops tea tree oil
15 drops peppermint oil
15 drops clove oil
5 to 10 drops neem oil

Blend these ingredients thoroughly and apply a few drops to the gums with a dropper or a cotton ball three times per day.

Tooth Powder Recipe for Pyorrhea

1 teaspoon finely ground bone meal
2 teaspoons ground cinnamon
4 teaspoons bentonite clay
1 teaspoon sea salt or other (high mineral natural salt)
2 drops food grade peppermint oil or a pinch of ground,

dried peppermint leaves
2 drops myrrh oil or a pinch of ground myrrh
1 teaspoon activated charcoal

Blend thoroughly in a blender or with a mortar and pestle.

References:

Nakamura R, Littarru GP, Folkers K, Wilkinson EG. Study of CoQ10-enzymes in gingiva from patients with periodontal disease and evidence for a deficiency of coenzyme Q10. Proc Natl. Acad Sci. 1974; 71:1456-1460.

5 OIL PULLING

Oil pulling is the common name for an ancient Ayurvedic healing and detoxifying technique from India. Traditionally, it is done using sesame seed or sunflower oils, but it can be successfully performed with almost any healthy, natural (preferably organic) oil.

Any of the following oils may be used:

Apricot
Castor
Coconut, preferably organic, virgin
Grape seed
Hemp seed
Olive

Take about a tablespoon of oil into your mouth and hold it there for 10 to 15 minutes. While you do this, swish it all around and force it in between your teeth. If you have an area of your mouth that is causing you particular concern or pain, allow the oil to saturate the area.

When the time has passed, spit the oil into the toilet. Optionally, you can rinse your mouth with warm sea salt water. Then drink plenty of fresh water (two or three glasses) to help facilitate the removal of toxins from your entire system.

It can be performed any time of day. It is ideal to do it in the morning before you have had any water to drink. If you want to detoxify more quickly, do oil pulling two or three times per day. Do not swallow the oil. If you happen to swallow a little of the oil and feel nauseated, place one or two drops of peppermint oil on your tongue or sip a little pineapple juice to quell the nausea.

Oil pulling can relieve some conditions in a matter of two or three days. It is a perfectly safe practice and one you should continue once per day or once per week, as you feel it is necessary, to maintain healthy teeth and gums.

6 HEALING CAVITIES AND CRACKED OR DAMAGED TEETH

Many people never look for a natural solution to the problem of cavities because they have been led to believe that once a cavity has formed, a tooth cannot be healed. But, it is possible to restore the enamel, re-mineralize and reinforce the health of your teeth with the proper nutrition and procedure.

During this process, the teeth must be kept scrupulously clean. Do not use glycerin-containing products, which coat the teeth and impede the process of re-mineralization.

One of the most powerful herbs for the re-mineralization of the teeth is horsetail (Equisetum arvense), also known as shave grass and colo de caballo. The stems of this plant contain a large amount of silica, which facilitates the absorption of calcium in the teeth. This plant is most efficacious when it is used fresh and the stems are chewed, but it is, also, very powerful when it is dried and chewed or used as a tooth powder. Look for the highest quality of organic horsetail you can find or, better yet, cultivate your own from seeds, which you can purchase and even trade for online.

If you have a problem tooth, one that is fractured, dark, broken or has a cavity, chew one to two teaspoons of horsetail, fresh or dried. The process of chewing helps get the silica into the saliva and is a superior method to simply swallowing the capsules. Do not take it for more than ten days at a time. Then take a break for, at least, three days.

Use a twig to stimulate your teeth. You can pull one from an oak tree, a dogwood tree, a cedar, a willow or any other tree and form a "toothbrush" out of it, with which you should scrub the surfaces of your teeth. Choose one about 1/4 inch diameter, peel back the bark and shape the end into an angle and rub your teeth with it. If you have a problem tooth, pay special attention to it when you rub it with the wood.

The twigs of the neem tree may be the most powerful for cleaning the teeth in this way. In its native India, the neem tree is called the "toothbrush tree" because it is used for all aspects of oral health. A number of neem suppliers online sell neem twigs (dentoon), neem oil and other neem-related oral care products.

You can also use miswak sticks, which come from the peelu tree and are commonly available in health food stores.

After eating, always brush your teeth with a healing tooth powder or paste that does not contain glycerin. (Tooth Powder Remedies are in Appendix A). Rub your teeth with the wood. If you have a cavity or other damaged tooth you are trying to heal, make a poultice of fresh or freshly dried horsetail by chewing it and packing it into the cavity of the tooth or hold it on the problem tooth with your tongue. Keep it there for as long as you can. It should be kept there constantly until the tooth is healed unless you are eating or cleaning your teeth.

By repeating this process of cleaning the teeth with an herbal tooth powder immediately after eating, followed by the rubbing of the teeth with a twig and then the application of a horsetail poultice on any tooth that is damaged, the teeth will begin to heal and the enamel will begin to restore itself over the damaged area of the tooth. This process may take days or weeks. Once your teeth are healed, you can maintain their mineral content and preserve your tooth enamel by reducing your chewing of horsetail to only two to three times per week.

As you go through this healing procedure for your teeth, continue to practice oil pulling up to three times per day.

Avoid processed foods and sugars, particularly during the healing period. Choose healthy, whole, organic, raw and unprocessed foods and fresh juices. Consume the healthy nutrients mentioned in earlier chapters and listed at the end of this book in "Appendix C."

Food grade diatomaceous Earth (DE) which is very high in silica can, also, be added to the diet to facilitate re-mineralization of sick or damaged teeth and the repair of tooth enamel. As a supplement, take one to two tablespoons per day.

Other silica-containing herbs and foods you can add to your diet:

Alfalfa
Buckwheat
Chickweed
Dandelions
Kelp
Lamb's quarters
Oat straw
Oats
Lentils

Raspberry leaf
Spelt
Sunflower seeds
Tomatoes

Include a supplement with trace minerals.

Another way to heal cavities and painful teeth is to combine equal parts of bentonite clay and activated charcoal. Make a paste with water and apply it to a decayed or painful tooth using your tongue to place the mixture inside the cavity. This remedy came from an unknown caller on the June 23, 2009 broadcast of the Officer Jack McLamb radio show at www.JackMcLamb.com. The caller claimed that it saved his teeth from unnecessary extractions and restored the health of his tooth. But, the clay and charcoal mixture is not to be used on a broken tooth because it can cause pain.

Try using the same bentonite clay and activated charcoal mixture in equal parts, but moisten it with a few drops of colloidal silver for extra antibiotic and healing effects.

You may see benefits from this overnight. It may, also, relieve tooth pain from the cavity. Continue using this mixture on the tooth, cleaning your teeth thoroughly after every meal and rubbing them with a healing neem twig or other type of twig, as described above, until the teeth are healed.

If you have a filling, it will have to be removed before you can grow enamel over the injured part of the tooth. Even if the filling remains in place, re-mineralization can still occur, which should strengthen the remaining part of the tooth.

Re-mineralization should not affect fillings. But, if a filling should come loose, you may then experiment with healing the tooth through the aforementioned procedure.

Mercury Amalgam Fillings

If you have or have ever had a "silver" mercury amalgam filling, then your body would probably benefit from a simple mercury detox. To perform a mercury detox, you need to get a little cilantro into your diet every day for, at least, two weeks.

Additionally, alfalfa, garlic, chlorella and fish oil help to chelate this toxic heavy metal from your system.

Juice a handful of cilantro, eat it in a salad or soup or enjoy one of these truly delicious recipes:

Fresh Cilantro Salsa

3 to 4 fresh tomatoes (medium to large)
Juice of one large fresh lime
1/2 large onion chopped
1 to 3 jalapeños (depending on how much heat you like)
Sea salt to taste
1/2 bunch or so of chopped cilantro

Chop the tomatoes and combine them with the lime juice in a blender. Add the onion and peppers. Then, add the salt to taste.

Blend this thoroughly. Add the cilantro last and then don't over-blend.

Your salsa should be a pretty, red color with flecks of green in it when you're finished. Serve immediately and refrigerate what you don't use.

Cilantro Pesto

1 to 3 peeled cloves of fresh garlic
1/2 cup almonds
1 cup (about 1 bunch) packed, fresh cilantro leaves
2 tablespoons lemon or lime juice
6 tablespoons olive oil
Sea salt to taste

Finely chop the fresh cilantro. Combine the ingredients in a blender and blend them until smooth and green.

Dr. David Williams published a similar Cilantro Pesto recipe in his newsletter, *Alternatives: For the Health Conscious Individual*, (Vol. 7, No. 12), June, 1998.

What to avoid:

De-mineralization occurs as a result of inadequate nutrition, radiation from x-rays, bacteria, processed sugar and processed grains. The metal instruments of dentists can cause injuries to teeth. So can bruxism (tooth grinding) and bad habits such as eating ice or hard candy. Avoid these things along with aspartame and other artificial sweeteners. Choose stevia, instead, because it is actually good for your teeth.

7 TMJ (LOCKJAW) AND BRUXISM (TOOTH GRINDING)

TMJ (Temporomandibular Joint Disorder) is, also, sometimes called "lockjaw." TMJ can have different causes. It may be caused by an infected tooth or an infection in the jaw, itself. Sometimes dentists are too rough with their patients, particularly children, pulling the jaw out of alignment. Some people acquire TMJ after a dental injection. In some cases, it can be caused by Tetanus.

But, very often it is simply the result of stress or pain in the teeth or elsewhere in the body. For example, if you experience sinus pain, you may experience a tightened jaw. TMJ can cause uncontrollable spasms causing you to hit your teeth together violently. It can even knock teeth loose.

If you believe your TMJ is caused by an oral infection, take the aforementioned steps to remedy it.

If you still suffer from TMJ after you have eliminated

bacterial causes, take your lifestyle into consideration. Ask yourself if your TMJ is the result of your stressful job, stressful relationships or other sources of negative stress. One of the most common causes of TMJ is stress.

TMJ is frequently accompanied by bruxism (tooth grinding). It can lead to damaged teeth and eroded enamel. Sometimes bruxism is so severe that it causes the enamel of the tooth to thin to the point of transparency. In such cases, follow the re-mineralization protocol above involving diet and horsetail to thicken the enamel.

If you have an acute case of TMJ or bruxism that is causing you to grind your teeth at night, you should consider a dental guard. You can purchase an inexpensive one at many pharmacies or you can be fitted for one at a dental office. If you have a dentist fit you with a guard, have one made that does not contain metal. If it clamps onto your teeth with metal, it will eventually wear or damage your teeth.

Try to relax your jaw during the day. Above all, keep your teeth from touching during the day and you will have better control at night. Also, change the posture of your tongue in your mouth, so that it reaches out to cover your lower teeth and prevents you from hitting them together. This feels strange at first, but after a few days, it becomes second nature and it will help to guard your teeth from blows and habitual grinding.

Meanwhile, there are some herbs you can use to reduce your stress and help your muscles relax. The most important of these is valerian root.

Valerian in whole root form, ground or powdered and drunk as a tea before bedtime will help all of the muscles of the body relax. The first night, the effect might not be dramatic, but by the second or third night of drinking this tea before bedtime, you should find yourself much more relaxed.

Valerian root has an unpleasant smell which can be mitigated by combining it with other relaxing herbs like lemon grass and chamomile. You can use tea bags or dried herbs. If you're using dried herbs, a pinch of each will do.

If you want to make these herbs even stronger and more powerful, decoct them. Simply let the water boil with the herbs and roots in it for a few minutes.

Use this tea or decoction as often as you like. But, be warned that it can produce a state of over-relaxation, if it is used for a long period of time. Drink it before bedtime or before a nap. Do not drink it right before driving a car or operating heavy machinery. Valerian root is not known to be toxic to people in good health.

People suffering from stress-related TMJ and bruxism should have good vitamin support, especially Vitamin B6, a Multi-B complex and magnesium. When the body is under stress, B vitamins are quickly depleted leaving you feeling less able to cope. Sufficient magnesium helps stop muscle spasms.

If you are under a great deal of stress, there is no herb or pill that can help you. Over a long period of time, sustained high levels of anxiety are damaging not only to your teeth, but your overall health. To stop the stress and possibly end your bruxism and TMJ, you must face the reality of your situation and make plans to change your lifestyle, if necessary. Sometimes, this is the only permanent solution.

8 NATURAL TOOTH WHITENING

Just as some foods and other substances can cause your teeth to yellow, there are foods, minerals and other substances that can whiten them. To whiten your teeth naturally, maintain a diet rich in Vitamin C along with any of the following remedies.

This tooth whitening remedy is widely attributed to Ben Franklin: Combine powdered charcoal and honey into a paste and apply it to the teeth.

Just brushing your teeth with a small amount of activated charcoal powder can whiten them after a couple of weeks. Although, brushing with charcoal can cause temporary darkening as the small flakes of charcoal get into tiny pores in the teeth. Keep brushing with charcoal and over time your teeth will become whiter and healthier.

Eating strawberries or crushing them and using the berries as a toothpaste is another common remedy for naturally white teeth. Do not rinse your mouth, but allow the strawberries to remain on your teeth for as long as possible.

One of the most popular and powerful natural whiteners is food grade hydrogen peroxide. It is, also, an effective anti-bacterial and it helps you to have an overall healthy mouth, naturally. Put a few drops of hydrogen peroxide on your toothbrush whenever you brush your teeth. You can, also, use diluted hydrogen peroxide as a tooth-whitening mouth rinse.

Rub your teeth with the twigs or powdered bark from the babul or banyan trees, both of which are native to India.

Add dried, powdered holy basil to your tooth powder for whitening.

Keep your teeth free of plaque. Add a tablespoon of vinegar to the reservoir of your oral irrigator.

Use a tea made of chaparral as a mouthwash to prevent the build up of plaque. Add a few drops of spearmint or peppermint oil to enhance its plaque-fighting power.

What to avoid: Coffee, black tea and smoking.

APPENDIX A
TOOTH POWDER REMEDIES

A reminder: When you use essential oils in oral applications, look for food grade oils and the highest quality you can find. Some essential oils labeled "100% essential oil" are highly diluted with essential oil of jojoba. Look for the highest grade of oils you can find.

Surprisingly good, food grade peppermint oil can be found in tiny one-dram bottles like those manufactured by Lorann Gourmet. For other oils, Eden Botanicals (www.edenbotanicals.com) is a good source. Before ordering an expensive oil, request a sample.

When you use these oils, you may want to start with half the number of drops recommended in the recipe and then add more only if it suits your tastes. You should go easy on the essential oils, at least, at first because some people are more sensitive to them than others. What is just right for one person might be too much for another.

Tooth powder recipes are not an exact science. You can adjust any of these recipes or make up your own. Use a single herb, like powdered cinnamon or powdered basil, if you like.

If you don't feel like making your own tooth powder, another alternative to commercial toothpaste is tooth soap. There are some small companies making and selling tooth soap flakes in a jar.

You can save money by just running your toothbrush across a bar of natural, organic soap, old-fashioned lye soap or Castille soap and brushing your teeth. Do not use glycerin soap or commercial soaps, which contain unnatural perfumes and harsh detergents.

For tooth powder recipes, use a blender or mortar and pestle to grind the ingredients together, bottle them in an air tight container. Dip your toothbrush into the mixture and brush your teeth.

Anti-gingivitis Sage & Myrrh Tooth Powder Recipes

1/4 cup ground sea salt
1/4 cup dried horsetail
1/4 cup dried sage leaves
1 tablespoon peppermint or spearmint leaves
10 drops myrrh oil or 1/4 teaspoon or so of myrrh powder

Gum Tightening Cinnamon Tooth Powder

1 tablespoon bentonite clay
2 tablespoons sea salt
1 tablespoon dried chaparral
2 teaspoons ground cinnamon

Purifying Peppermint Tooth Powder

1 cup food grade calcium carbonate
2 tablespoons bentonite clay
1 tablespoon powdered lye or pure Castille soap
5 drops clove oil
15 drops food grade peppermint oil

APPENDIX B
MOUTHWASH REMEDIES

You can use similar creativity with your mouth washes as you do with tooth powders. Examples of good liquid bases are vodka (other pure grain alcohol or brandy), colloidal silver and clean water. You may combine tinctures and oils into your mouthwashes. Bottle them and shake them well before using them.

Healing Mouthwash

1 cup echinacea tea
2 ounces vodka
5 to 10 drops cinnamon oil

Refreshing Anti-bacterial Mouthwash

2 tablespoons vodka
1 cup colloidal silver
3 drops tea tree oil
5 drops peppermint oil

Soothing Mouthwash

1 tablespoon bicarbonate of soda
1 tablespoon sea salt
2 cups water
2 tablespoons colloidal silver (optional)

Anti-gingivitis Mouthwash

1 cup myrrh tea
1 cup colloidal silver
1 tablespoon vodka
5 drops cinnamon oil
1 cup chaparral tea
1 cup echinacea tea
5 to 10 drops clove oil

APPENDIX C
LIST OF DENTAL HEALING AGENTS

Minerals

Activated charcoal (healing and whitening)
Bone meal
Calcium
Colloidal silver (pure)
Diatomaceous earth
Dolomite
Fulvic minerals
Magnesium
Phosphorus

Trace Elements

Boron
Copper
Iodine
Fluorine
Zinc

Vitamins

Bioflavinoids (Vitamin P)
B-Complex
B12
C (natural sources - do not chew)
D
E (natural sources)
Folic acid
K, especially K2
Niacin

Herbs and Fruits and Vegetables

Alfalfa leaf
Aloe vera
Amla (decoction for strengthening teeth)
Alum
Anise
Bilberry
Cardamom (bad breath)
Calamus
Calendula
Chaparral
Chlorophyll (gums and bad breath)
Cinnamon
Comfrey (compresses for pain)
Echinacea
Garlic
Hawthorn berry
Holy basil
Horsetail
Irish moss
Juniper
Kelp

Lobelia hypopnea (dental pain)
Myrrh
Neem
Onion
Orris root (whitening)
Plantain
Prickly pear
Red dock
Rosemary
Sage (particularly white sage)
Strawberries
Tarragon
Turmeric root
Valerian
Vanilla extract
Wheat grass juice
Wild lettuce (dental pain)
Yellow dock root
The juice of all leafy greens.

Essential Oils

Cajeput
Caraway
Chamomile
Clove
Eucalyptus
Oregano
Peppermint
Tea tree
Thyme
Wheat germ

Vegetable and Fruit Oils Used in Oil Pulling

Apricot
Castor
Coconut
Hemp seed
Olive
Sesame
Sunflower (whitening)

Wood

Babul bark (whitening)
Banyan (whitening)
Cinchona bark
Goldenseal root
Miswak sticks from the peelu tree
Neem twigs
Oak bark
Prickly ash bark
Wood ash

Mercury Chelation Herbs and Supplements

Alfalfa
Cilantro
Chlorella
Fish oil
Garlic

Miscellaneous

Cod liver oil
CoQ10
Honey

Hydrogen peroxide
Propolis
Sea salt
Soap (pure Castille or lye soap - run your toothbrush across it and brush your teeth)

To Avoid or Limit

Acidic foods and beverages like coffee, black tea and sodas
Lemon juice (erodes enamel and causes sensitivity)
Processed grains

OTHER WINTER TEMPEST BOOKS

If you enjoyed this book, you might enjoy other Winter Tempest Books:

Magical Healing: How to Use Your Mind to Heal Yourself and Others by Angela Kaelin

Natural Remedies for Reversing Gray Hair: Nutrition and Herbs for Anti-aging and Optimum Health by Thomas W. Xander

Traditional Witches' Formulary and Potion-making Guide: Recipes for Magical Oils, Powders and Other Potions by Sophia diGregorio

Legal Disclaimer: The author and publisher of this guide has used her best efforts in preparing this document. The author makes no representation or warranties with respect to the accuracy, applicability, fitness or completeness of the contents of this document. The author disclaims any warranties expressed or implied. Nothing in this document should be construed as medical advice. The author shall in no event be held liable for any loss or damages, including but not limited to special, incidental, consequential or other damages incurred by the use of this information. The statements in this book have not been evaluated by the F.D.A., the A.M.A., the A.D.A. or any other government organization. The statements contained herein represent the legally protected opinions of the author and are presented for informational purposes only. If anyone uses any of this information in the book, they do so at their own risk. This document contains material protected under copyright laws. Any unauthorized reprint, transmission or resale of this material without the express permission of the author is strictly prohibited.

FTC Disclaimer: The author has no connection to nor was paid by any brand or product described in this document except for Winter Tempest Books.

FDA Disclaimer: The statements in this book are the opinion of the author and have not been evaluated by the Food and Drug Administration. Products and information provided on this site are not intended to diagnose, treat, cure or prevent any disease. If you have a medical condition, consult your physician. All information is provided for educational purposes only. Please consult your doctor if your pregnant. Keep these and all supplements out of the reach of children.

30268949R00033

Made in the USA
Lexington, KY
25 February 2014